Vaccine Victories

The Parent's Guide to Immunizations

Table of Contents

Chapter 1. Introduction

Navigating the world of vaccinations can feel like steering through an overwhelming sea of information. In our special report, "Vaccine Victories: The Parent's Guide to Immunizations," we simplify this critical journey for you. We've researched extensively, consulted with healthcare professionals, and have compiled data from trusted sources around the globe to present a comprehensive, parent-friendly guide. Within this report, you'll find easy-to-understand explanations, debunked myths, as well as data-backed benefits of vaccines, ensuring your child grows up healthy and protected. So whether you're a new parent or need a quick refresher, our special report emerges as your trusty lighthouse amidst the waves of vaccine-related worries. Enjoy this empowering journey to responsible parenthood, because every child deserves a shot at a healthy future!

Chapter 2. Understanding the Basics: What Vaccines Are and How They Work

One of the first steps towards comprehending the world of vaccines is understanding what they are and how they function. In essence, vaccines are substances that stimulate the body's immune system to recognize and fight specific viruses or bacteria. The process of vaccination trains the body to combat these infectious agents without causing the disease itself.

2.1. The Basic Components of Vaccines

There are several types of vaccines, each composed of different components. However, all vaccines consist of some critical pieces:

- Antigen: This is the element of the vaccine that our bodies recognize as an invader. Antigens are often harmless versions or parts of the viruses or bacteria that they are designed to protect against. They could be live but weakened forms of the pathogen (as used in measles or mumps vaccines), killed or inactivated versions (as in the polio vaccine), or fragments of the pathogen like its protein or sugar.

- Adjuvants: These are substances that help boost the body's response to the vaccine. They stimulate the immune system, ensuring that the vaccine is more effective.

- Stabilizers: These protect the vaccine from changing or degrading over time. They ensure the vaccine remains effective during storage and transportation.

- Preservatives: These prevent the growth of bacteria or fungi in the vaccine, particularly in multi-dose vials from which multiple doses are drawn.

Please note that contrary to some misconceptions, vaccines do not contain harmful levels of toxins. The components of vaccines, including trace amounts of potential toxins, are carefully monitored and controlled to ensure safety.

2.2. Working Principle of Vaccines

When you receive a vaccine, your immune system springs into action. It does not matter whether the vaccine was injected, ingested orally, or administered nasally. The immune responses generally follow these steps:

1. Pathogen Recognition: The immune cells, primarily B and T lymphocytes, identify the antigen as foreign.

2. Immune Response and Memory Cell Creation: The immune system mounts a defense involving several types of white blood cells. B-cells produce antibodies that latch onto the antigens to neutralize them or mark them for destruction, while T-cells destroy the infected cells. Importantly, the immune system also creates specific memory cells during this process.

3. Future Exposure: If you ever encounter the actual disease-causing pathogen, your immune system is prepared. The memory cells recognize the invader and initiate a faster and stronger immune response.

2.3. Vaccination Schedule

There is a specific schedule of vaccination that is recommended for different age groups, especially infants and children. This schedule is designed to offer protection when children are most vulnerable and before they are potentially exposed to diseases. Vaccination schedules can vary slightly by country, but they generally follow the World Health Organization (WHO) guidelines. Always discuss the schedule with your healthcare professional.

2.4. The Benefits of Vaccines

Vaccination goes beyond personal health protection. The widespread use of vaccines can contribute to 'herd immunity,' a state where a sufficient percentage of the population is immune to a disease, reducing its spread and even potentially eradicating it.

Herd immunity provides indirect protection to those who can't be vaccinated, such as infants, pregnant women, or immunocompromised individuals. Diseases like smallpox and rinderpest have been eradicated thanks to vaccination, and polio is on the brink of eradication.

In conclusion, understanding vaccines and their function is crucial for comprehending their role in public health and personal wellbeing. Vaccines train our immune systems to fend off harmful pathogens without exposing us to the risks associated with the diseases they cause. With regular vaccinations as per recommended schedules, we can ensure our individual health and contribute to the larger goal of disease control and elimination, making our world a healthier place.

Chapter 3. The Full Schedule: A Chronological Guide to Immunizations

Keeping an organized schedule for your child's vaccinations can seem daunting. However, the process becomes more manageable when you understand each vaccine's purpose and timing. In this section, we delve deep into the chronological guide of immunizations, helping you keep track from birth to the teenage years.

3.1. Birth to 6 months

Within the first 6 months, your little one will receive a series of vaccines:

1. Hepatitis B vaccine (HepB): Given at birth, the HepB vaccine protects against the hepatitis B virus that can cause severe liver diseases. A second dose follows at 1–2 months, and a third dose at 6–18 months.

2. DTaP: This vaccine, administered at 2 months, 4 months, and 6 months, shields against Diphtheria, Tetanus, and Pertussis (whooping cough).

3. Hib (Haemophilus influenzae type b): Given at the same periods as DTaP, the Hib vaccine prevents diseases caused by Haemophilus influenza type b bacteria.

4. Polio vaccine (IPV): First dose at 2 months, with follow-ups at 4 months and 6–18 months, IPV safeguards against polio.

5. Pneumococcal vaccine (PCV): Administered at the 2nd, 4th, and 6th months, PCV protects from pneumococcal diseases like pneumonia.

6. Rotavirus vaccine (RV): RV, given at 2 and 4 months, is your child's defense against the rotavirus causing severe diarrhea in babies.

3.2. 7 to 18 months

This period introduces some vaccines and continues the doses started earlier:

1. DTaP: Your baby will receive a fourth dose anytime between 15-18 months.

2. Hib: The fourth and final dose of Hib is administered between 12-15 months.

3. PCV: The final dose is also given between 12-15 months.

4. IPV: A booster is given between 6-18 months.

5. HepB: The third and final dose is delivered between 6-18 months.

6. Measles, Mumps, and Rubella (MMR): The first dose is typically administered at 12-15 months.

7. Varicella (Chickenpox): The initial dose is given within the same window as the MMR.

8. Hepatitis A: Your child will receive the first of two doses between 12-23 months. Within 6 to 18 months of the first dose, the second dose is given.

3.3. 19 months to 4 years

The emphasis during this age window is on booster vaccinations:

1. DTaP: The fifth dose, or booster, usually occurs between 4-6 years.

2. Polio (IPV): The fourth and final dose is administered at 4-6 years.

3.4. 4 to 6 years

This phase is typically lighter with immunizations involving only boosters:

1. MMR: An MMR booster is given between 4–6 years.

2. Varicella: Similar to MMR, a booster is given between 4-6 years.

3.5. 7 to 18 years

As your child grows into an adolescent, few more vaccines are added:

1. Human Papillomavirus vaccine (HPV): It's recommended at 11-12 years, but can start as early as 9 years and as late as 26. The vaccine is typically given in two doses, 6-12 months apart.

2. Tetanus, Diphtheria, and Pertussis (Tdap): As a part of continuing protection, Tdap is provided at 11-12 years.

3. Meningococcal vaccines: These vaccines (MenACWY-D, MenACWY-CRM, MenB-FHbp, and MenB-4C) protect against meningococcal diseases, usually given at 11-12 years and a booster at 16 years.

Immunization is a significant step in guaranteeing your child's health and safety. This chronological guide should aid you in effectively tracking your child's vaccine schedule. However, changes to vaccination schedules can occur based on updated research and local health advisories. It is essential to consult with your healthcare provider regularly to understand the best course of action for your child's immunizations.

In our next chapter, we move towards discussing how vaccines work, their safety, efficacy, and common misconceptions to further equip you with the knowledge necessary for your child's wellness journey.

Chapter 4. Benefits of Vaccinations: Safeguarding Your Child's Health

An introduction to vaccinations may combat a crucial foe: infectious diseases. For centuries, these formidable adversaries have wreaked havoc on the health of children and adults alike. The advent of vaccinations has turned the tide in this ongoing battle, significantly decreasing, and in some cases completely eradicating, the incidence of certain diseases.

4.1. Understanding the Role of Vaccinations

Vaccines play an essential role in protecting your child's health by boosting their immune system to fight off potentially harmful pathogens. Their primary function is to teach the immune system to recognize and combat specific viruses and bacteria, equipping it with the knowledge it needs to nip threats in the bud.

The process involves the introduction of inactive or weakened strains of a particular pathogen to stimulate the immune system's response without causing the full-blown disease. This exposure allows the body to safely produce the required antibodies to counter the pathogen and store that information for future encounters.

4.2. The Shield Against a Plethora of Diseases

From measles, mumps, and polio to influenza and Hepatitis B, vaccines are designed to protect against a broad array of diseases.

These particular illnesses, while less common now thanks to vaccinations, can result in serious, life-threatening complications, particularly in children.

For instance, measles can lead to brain swelling and permanent damage, not to mention death in severe cases. Polio, while eradicated in many parts of the world, still surfaces sporadically and can cause permanent paralysis.

Similarly, bacterial pathogens can cause illnesses such as meningitis and pneumonia, both of which can be deadly if not treated immediately. Vaccines provide an effective shield against these and more unseen enemies, helping your child live a healthier life.

4.3. Herd Immunity: A Shared Responsibility

Another vital reason for immunizing children is to promote herd immunity, a concept where a significantly high percentage of a population receiving vaccinations can also protect those who can't get vaccinated due to medical conditions or age.

By ensuring your child gets vaccinated, you are playing a crucial role in achieving and maintaining this shield of immunity for the community. Herd immunity is vital, especially for infants who are too young to receive certain vaccines and people with weakened immune systems due to illness or treatments such as chemotherapy.

4.4. Dealing with the 'Vaccines and Autism' Myth

One of the most pervasive myths about vaccinations is their alleged link to autism. This misconception was born out of a study published in 1998 that has since been not only debunked but also retracted due to serious procedural errors and ethical violations.

Multiple studies involving millions of children worldwide have found no link between vaccines and autism. The Centers for Disease Control and Prevention (CDC), World Health Organization (WHO), and the Institute of Medicine (IOM) are among the reputable institutes that uniformly assert the safety and necessity of vaccines.

4.5. The Statistical Strength of Vaccines

In a measurable context, vaccines have accomplished remarkable feats in disease control. Consider this: before the measles vaccine was introduced in 1963, millions of cases occurred each year in the United States. By 2000, due to vaccination efforts, measles was declared eliminated from the country.

Another example is polio - once a feared disease causing paralysis and death, it's now a memory in many parts of the world, thanks to the polio vaccine. The Global Polio Eradication Initiative reports a decrease in polio cases by over 99% since 1988.

4.6. Vaccines: The Cost-Efficient Way for Health Protection

Beyond the health benefits, vaccinations offer a cost-effective way to guard against diseases. The price of getting vaccinations is lower compared to the expenses incurred in treating the diseases they prevent, which often involve hospitalizations and long-term care.

Besides, several insurance plans cover the cost of vaccinations, and public programs like the Vaccines for Children (VFC) Program provides vaccines free of charge to eligible children.

Ensuring your child receives the full course of recommended vaccinations is an investment in their long-term health. This proactive approach will shield them and others around them from serious diseases and yield a stronger, healthier community. It might seem like a lot to navigate, but with each vaccination, we take one step closer to a healthier future for our children.

Chapter 5. A Closer Look: The Science Behind Vaccine Safety

The journey to understanding vaccine safety begins by recognizing the incredible scientific processes that lie behind every dose administered. A vaccine's life starts in a research lab, moves through rigorous phases of testing, and continues to be monitored even after its public release.

5.1. The Building Blocks of Vaccines

Vaccines work because they mimic the infection-causing pathogens that invade our bodies. These disease-causing agents stimulate our immune system, which responds by creating weapons in the form of antibodies to fight these intruders. The genius of a vaccine is that it replicates this process without us having to suffer through the actual disease.

To stimulate an immune response, vaccines contain ingredients like antigens, adjuvants, and stabilizers. Antigens are weakened or inactive versions of the disease-causing pathogens, or even fragments of these organisms. Adjuvants amplify the immune response, while stabilizers ensure the vaccine remains effective during its shelf-life.

In addition to these, vaccines may also contain trace amounts of substances used during the production process, such as formaldehyde or antibiotics, to ensure the final product is safe and effective. While these names might sound alarming, the quantities involved are tiny, and their safety has been well-established through substantial research.

5.2. The Rigorous Development Process

Before it is administered to people, a vaccine undergoes rigorous testing during development. This process often takes many years, if not decades, and involves several critical stages.

Preclinical trials pave the way. During these, the vaccine candidate is tested in a laboratory and on animals to evaluate safety and the ability to provoke an immune response. After promising results from preclinical trials, the candidate moves on to Phase I clinical trials where a small group of volunteers (often healthy adults) are administered the vaccine. Here, researchers evaluate its safety, determine the right dose, and identify any side-effects.

Phase II involves a slightly larger group of volunteers, including those similar to the people for whom the vaccine is intended. Here, the vaccine's safety, immunogenicity (ability to provoke an immune response), and potential side effects are further investigated.

Phase III trials increase the participant pool to thousands and allow researchers to identify any rare side effects that might not have been evident in smaller groups. It also helps ascertain the vaccine's effectiveness and how it performs across different demographics.

Only after successfully passing these phases does a vaccine receive approval from the relevant health authorities, such as the Food and Drug Administration in the US. But approval is not the end; the vaccine continues to be scrutinized in the next stage - post-marketing surveillance.

5.3. Post-Marketing Surveillance: Ensuring Continued Safety

Post-marketing surveillance monitors the vaccine's safety and performance even after it has been approved. Health authorities regularly review reports of potential side effects (also known as adverse events). This ongoing monitoring provides an opportunity to identify rare side effects that may only occur in very large populations or specific demographic groups.

Tools like the Vaccine Adverse Event Reporting System (VAERS) in the US and the Yellow Card Scheme in the UK are essential for this process. Everyone — including healthcare professionals, vaccine manufacturers, and the public — can use these systems to report suspected side effects.

Two other systems deployed in the US are the Vaccine Safety Datalink and the Clinical Immunization Safety Assessment Network, which allow for active surveillance and timely evaluation of potential vaccine safety issues. Globally, the use of such monitoring systems ensures that even the rarest of side effects is not missed.

5.4. A Case Study: The COVID-19 Vaccines

For a real-world example of these principles in action, let's take a closer look at the development and post-market surveillance of the COVID-19 vaccines.

In response to the global pandemic, researchers worldwide have leveraged years of previous research on related coronaviruses like SARS and MERS to expedite the development of COVID-19 vaccines. Modern technologies such as mRNA have been employed to develop efficient and safe vaccines in a record time frame.

Despite the swift development, these vaccines have gone through the same stringent testing processes typical of any vaccine. The results from each phase of the clinical trials have been documented, reviewed, and published, and their safety continues to be monitored worldwide.

Should an issue arise with any vaccine, mechanisms exist to pause distribution, examine the data, and determine the best path forward. This process was used when health organizations temporarily halted the Johnson & Johnson COVID-19 vaccine's distribution to investigate a small number of cases of rare but severe types of blood clots.

The science behind vaccines, while complex, is guided by a single principle – protection of public health. With the evidence and systems at hand, we have every reason to trust that vaccines are safe and will continue to be our reliable allies in the fight against devastating diseases. It's important to make decisions about immunization based on accurate, up-to-date knowledge. By understanding the science behind vaccine safety, we can all contribute to healthier communities, safer environments for our children, and ultimately, a healthier future.

Chapter 6. Breaking Down the Misconceptions: Debunking Common Vaccine Myths

With so much information and, unfortunately, misinformation available about vaccines, it's easy to feel confused or overwhelmed. To help you distinguish fact from fiction, let's systematically debunk some common myths surrounding vaccines.

6.1. Vaccines and Autism Link

The most persistent misconception is that vaccines, particularly the MMR (Measles, Mumps, and Rubella) vaccine, are linked to autism. This claim originated from a 1998 study by Andrew Wakefield. However, several robust studies have found no connection between vaccines and autism.

The original 1998 study was severely flawed and later retracted. Wakefield, the lead researcher, lost his medical license due to ethical concerns around the study. Today, scientific consensus refutes any such link between vaccines and autism. According to the Centers for Disease Control and Prevention (CDC), multiple studies have confirmed that vaccines do not increase the risk of autism.

6.2. Too Many Vaccines Overwhelm the Immune System

Another commonly propagated myth is that being vaccinated with multiple vaccines can overwhelm a child's immune system. This stems from an understandable concern — after all, we want to protect our children from undue harm.

However, the idea that vaccines overload the immune system is unfounded. From birth, we encounter millions of microbes daily that our immune systems have to fight off. According to the World Health Organization (WHO), vaccines use a tiny fraction of the immune system's memory, leaving the vast majority of it available to combat other diseases.

Moreover, combination vaccines have been in use for many years and have a proven safety record. They allow for fewer injections and less discomfort for the child while ensuring adequate protection against dangerous diseases.

6.3. Natural Infection Is Better Than Vaccination

Some argue that it's better to get a disease naturally than to prevent it with a vaccine. While it's true that natural infection often leads to stronger immunity than vaccines, the risks far outweigh the benefits.

For example, catching measles naturally can result in serious complications, like pneumonia or brain swelling, which can lead to death. Vaccines, on the other hand, provide a safer and controlled way to gain immunity, without the health risks associated with the disease itself.

6.4. Vaccines Contain Harmful Ingredients

Many people worry about the ingredients used in vaccines. Common concerns include the presence of substances like mercury, formaldehyde, and aluminum.

It's important to note that components used in vaccines are safe in the amounts given. Thimerosal, a mercury-based preservative, has been verified as safe by numerous studies and is only used in a few vaccines. Moreover, our bodies naturally produce and metabolize formaldehyde, and the amounts found in vaccines are much smaller than already present in our system. As for aluminum, it boosts the vaccine's effectiveness and is eliminated by our kidneys.

6.5. Vaccines Are Not Needed Because Disease Rates Are Already Down

Some consider vaccines unnecessary because disease rates have decreased. This thinking is a product of vaccines' success — many people in industrialized countries have never seen the diseases vaccines prevent. As a result, they underestimate the seriousness of these diseases and the importance of immunization.

Vaccines have dramatically reduced, and in some cases, eradicated diseases that were once widespread. But just because a disease is currently rare, it doesn't mean it can't return. If vaccination rates drop, these diseases could make a comeback.

6.6. Vaccines Are Not Tested Enough

Lastly, there's a myth that vaccines are not tested rigorously. In reality, vaccines are among the most tested medical interventions, subjected to numerous trials before approval and continually monitored for safety after rollout. Both national and international health organizations keep a close eye on vaccine safety, ensuring that they remain effective and any side effects are quickly identified.

In conclusion, vaccinations are a crucial part of ensuring your child's health and the health of their community. As you navigate your own journey through the world of vaccines, always seek advice from reliable and credible resources. Proper information is the first step towards safeguarding our children's future.

Chapter 7. Addressing Concerns: Side Effects and How to Handle Them

With the widespread awareness and availability of vaccines, you, as a parent, might have questions and concerns about their side effects and how to manage them. Addressing these concerns is vital to shaping a clear and informed perspective on vaccinations and their impact.

7.1. Understanding Side Effects

Side effects or adverse reactions from vaccines vary considerably from one individual to another, and most can be classified as minor. Most occur due to the body's natural response to foreign substances.

Minor vaccine side effects can include:

- Pain, swelling, or redness at the injection site

- Mild fever

- Tiredness

- Headache

- Muscle or joint pain

- Chills

- Nausea

These side effects are typically short-lived and can be managed effectively at home with simple interventions.

7.2. Dissecting Vaccine Ingredients

Vaccines contain various active ingredients that stimulate the body's immune system to develop protection against specific diseases. Here are the key ingredients found in vaccines:

- **Antigens**: These are weakened or inactivated forms of the virus or bacteria against which the vaccine offers protection.

- **Adjuvants**: These substances enhance the body's immune response to the antigen.

- **Preservatives**: These substances prevent contamination by bacteria or fungi.

- **Stabilizers**: These substances maintain vaccine potency during storage and transport.

- **Residuals**: Small amounts of substances used during production processes, such as cell culture materials, antibiotics, or inactivating ingredients, may remain as residuals in the vaccine.

Each ingredient plays a pivotal role in making vaccines efficacious and safe. The quantity of these ingredients is strictly regulated and remains well within safe limits.

7.3. Handling Common Side Effects at Home

Here are simple and effective ways to handle common side effects at home:

- For redness, swelling, or pain at the injection site: Use a clean, cool, wet cloth on the area. Over-the-counter medicine may be used under the guidance of a healthcare professional.

- For fever or discomfort: Ensure your child drinks plenty of fluids and dresses lightly. Over-the-counter fever reducers or pain relievers can sometimes be suggested by your child's healthcare provider.

- For general discomfort or unsettled mood: Provide plenty of rest, comfort, and assurance to your child.

It's crucial to stay in touch with the healthcare provider if any concern or discomfort persists beyond 48 hours or if new symptoms develop.

7.4. Rare Severe Side Effects

While severe side effects are rare, they are possible. Signs of severe allergic reactions may include:

- Difficulty breathing

- Hoarseness or wheezing

- Swelling around the eyes or lips

- Hives

- Paleness

- Weakness

- Rapid heart rate

- Feeling dizzy

If your child shows any signs of severe reactions, immediately seek emergency medical attention.

7.5. Vaccine Safety Monitoring

Post-marketing surveillance is a cornerstone of vaccine safety, conducted by international agencies like the WHO, the CDC in the US, and the MHRA in the UK. These bodies routinely collect, analyze, and interpret health-related data post-vaccination, enabling them to detect, verify, assess and investigate potential adverse events.

Parents should report any adverse events following immunization to their healthcare provider, who will then be able to forward the information to the relevant authorities.

7.6. Understanding Vaccine Myths and Realities

Myth: **Vaccines cause autism.** Reality: Studies have shown conclusively that there is no link between receiving vaccines and developing Autism Spectrum Disorder (ASD).

Myth: **Natural immunity is better than vaccine-acquired immunity.** Reality: While natural infections can provide immunity, the risks far outweigh the benefits. Vaccines induce immunity without causing illness.

Myth: **Vaccines contain harmful ingredients.** Reality: Vaccines contain ingredients that are safe for humans when administered in the approved quantities.

Vaccines are a critical part of your child's health care, and understanding vaccine side effects and their management is just as essential. A collaborative approach involving parents and healthcare professionals is necessary for successful and safe routine immunization. After all, protecting our children from preventable diseases is a shared responsibility.

Chapter 8. Beyond the Basics: Vaccine Efficiency and Herd Immunity

The process of vaccination serves as an essential line of defense in protecting our societies from debilitating or even deadly infectious diseases. More than just safeguarding an individual, vaccines play a crucial role in preserving the health of entire communities through a phenomenon known as 'herd immunity'. To fully appreciate the effectiveness of vaccines and the value of herd immunity, we must delve into the principles beyond basic immunization theories.

8.1. Understanding Vaccines

A vaccine works by training the body's immune system to recognize and combat pathogens, either viruses or bacteria. To accomplish this, certain molecules from the pathogen must be introduced into the body to trigger an immune response.

These molecules are called antigens, and they are contained in vaccines either live, attenuated (weakened), or inactivated forms of the pathogen, or in subunit compositions, that is, pieces of the disease-causing organism. When the immune system confronts these harmless antigens, it responds by producing molecules known as antibodies.

Upon exposure to the antigens contained in a vaccine, our bodies store information about those specific pathogens and how to defeat them. Later, if the organism ever invades our bodies, our immune system swiftly recognizes the invaders and rapidly produces the antibodies needed to fight them.

8.2. Efficacy of Vaccines

Vaccines have proven to be one of the most effective tools in preventing the spread of infectious diseases. Their efficacy can be measured in a couple of ways. Protection can be evaluated by measuring disease rates in a vaccinated population and comparing it to those in an unvaccinated population. Efficacy can also be estimated by examining the number of antibodies produced after vaccination.

Not all vaccines provide complete immunity – varying depending on the vaccine and illness. Despite this, the vast majority reduce the severity of diseases, deaths, and disease-specific complications significantly.

One remarkable vaccination success story is the eradication of smallpox. Due to extensive global vaccination campaigns, the last natural case of smallpox occurred in 1977.

8.3. Herd Immunity: The Basics and Beyond

Herd immunity, also known as community immunity, is a form of indirect protection from infectious disease that occurs when a large percentage of a population has become immune to an infection, thereby providing a measure of protection for individuals who are not immune.

For herd immunity to work, a certain threshold must be reached. This threshold depends on the contagiousness of the disease. Measles, for example, requires about 95% of a population to be vaccinated, while polio, mumps, and pertussis require about 80-85%.

Numerous studies have shown and continue to show the effectiveness of herd immunity in disease prevention. Its success, however, relies heavily on high rates of vaccine coverage. Without sustained vaccination rates, protection dwindles and diseases can rapidly re-emerge.

8.4. Herd Immunity and Children

Children, due to their growing immune systems, can be particularly susceptible to infectious diseases. Vaccinating children at the recommended ages allows them to build immunity before they are exposed to potentially life-threatening diseases.

It is important to note that some children cannot receive certain vaccinations due to severe allergies, weakened immune systems and other health-related issues. For these children, the only line of defense against certain diseases is the herd immunity that results from the immunization of others.

8.5. The Role of Vaccination in Achieving Herd Immunity

The key driver to achieving herd immunity is vaccination. Immunizations not only protect individuals but also block the spread of diseases within communities and even globally. The persistent efforts worldwide to immunize children have led to dramatic decreases in illnesses and deaths from diseases such as measles, whooping cough, and flu.

The journey toward achieving herd immunity requires collective action. Everyone who can get vaccinated not only protects themselves, but also helps prevent the spread of diseases throughout the community.

8.6. Breakthroughs and Challenges

The ongoing research involving vaccinations has led to significant breakthroughs in combating once-prevalent diseases. Nevertheless, numerous challenges persist, including vaccination hesitancy or refusal, public perception, and supply issues. Ensuring the efficient distribution of vaccines and sustaining vaccination rates is paramount.

Amidst these challenges, the importance of immunization and herd immunity cannot be overstated. They offer robust protections against diseases for individuals incapable of vaccination, enhance the overall health of communities, and show promise in completely eradicating some of humanity's most formidable infectious diseases.

By deepening our understanding of vaccines and herd immunity, we can better appreciate just how vital these tools are in our fight against infectious diseases. We owe it to our children, and indeed to all of society, to maintain a commitment to vaccination and aim for a healthier future.

Chapter 9. Special Circumstances: Vaccination for Children with Allergies and Immune Disorders

Vaccinating a child with allergies or immune disorders requires an understanding of both, the child's specific condition as well as the vaccine in question. While in some cases, allergies or immunity issues can complicate the immunization schedule, often times they do not pose an insurmountable challenge. As parent navigators, let us delve into this complex area.

9.1. Allergies and Vaccines

For the majority of children with common allergies, vaccination proceeds as usual. However, there are exceptions for children with specific severs allergies to vaccine components.

Let's begin by saying that the occurrence of severe allergic reactions to vaccines, also known as anaphylaxis, is extremely rare. The Centers for Disease Control and Prevention (CDC) puts this number at about one in a million. With this in mind, it's important to understand that vaccines have various components, and only a small number of them are typically associated with allergies.

Common allergenic substances in vaccines include egg protein (found in some influenza vaccines), gelatin (used as a stabilizer in some vaccines), and yeast (a component of the hepatitis B and HPV vaccines).

When a child has a known severe allergy to one of these substances, the doctor might choose an alternative vaccine that does not contain the allergenic substance. For example, there are several influenza vaccines that do not contain egg protein.

9.2. Immune Disorders and Vaccines

Moving to the consideration of immune disorders, the concern arises from the fact that vaccines are designed to stimulate the immune system. If a child has an immune system disorder, the response to a vaccine can be unpredictable.

There are two main types of vaccines: live-attenuated and inactivated vaccines. Live-attenuated vaccines contain a version of the living virus or bacteria that has been weakened so it cannot cause disease in people with healthy immune systems. Inactivated vaccines, on the other hand, are made from viruses or bacteria that have been killed or inactivated.

Children with immune disorders should generally not receive live-attenuated vaccines because there is a risk, albeit small, that the vaccine could cause disease. Inactivated vaccines, meanwhile, are generally safe for children with immune disorders. But they may not provoke a strong immune response, which means the vaccine might not be as effective as it would be in a child with a fully functioning immune system.

9.2.1. Vaccinating Children with Specific Immune Disorders

Depending on the nature of the immune disorder, some vaccines may be especially recommended, while others might be avoided. Here are a few examples:

- Children with HIV: Unless their immune system is severely compromised, children with HIV should receive most routine childhood vaccines. But, in general, they should avoid live-attenuated vaccines.

- For children who have received bone marrow transplants: These children often lose their immunity to diseases for which they were previously vaccinated. Post-transplant, they should generally be revaccinated with inactivated vaccines. However, they should wait at least three to six months post-transplant to start their vaccinations.

- Children who are receiving long-term steroids: These children may receive inactivated vaccines, but live-attenuated vaccines should be avoided.

9.3. Precautions and Proceeding Safely

Before any vaccination, let your healthcare provider know about any known allergies or immune disorders your child has. They will guide you with the potential risks and modifications to the immunization schedule if necessary.

Remember, the purpose of vaccinations is to prevent serious illnesses. While this requires understanding and managing risks, potential side effects should be weighed against the benefits of protecting your child from potentially deadly diseases.

Ultimately, the decision to vaccinate a child with allergies or immune disorders should be made in collaboration with healthcare professionals who know the child and understand their specific health situation. Their informed advice will ensure you are making the safe and healthy choices for your child, in light of their unique circumstances.

Chapter 10. Your Role: The Importance of Parental Consent in Immunization

In the journey of parenthood, informed decisions make an enormous difference in securing your child's health and future. The subject of immunization demands particular attention—taking full charge includes understanding why your consent is crucial and learning how to give informed consent.

10.1. Why Your Consent Matters

Immunization programs are grounded in a principle that rests upon two pillars: the wellbeing of the community and the autonomy of the individual. By consenting to your child's immunization, you are simultaneously contributing to achieving herd immunity—an indispensable social tool to stymie infectious diseases.

Note that, while benign, vaccines do introduce an external substance into the body. Therefore, gaining your fully aware consent—ensuring you understand the justification, potential risks, and benefits—is ethically indispensable.

As a parent, your informed consent signifies that you:

1. Understand the purpose of the vaccines.

2. Comprehend the potential benefits and risks.

3. Are aware of the alternative courses of action, including non-immunization.

4. Have had opportunities to ask questions and are satisfied with the answers.

10.2. Informed Consent: An Ethical Imperative

Informed consent goes beyond signing a paper—it's an ethical and legal prerequisite in the medical field, aimed at protecting an individual's autonomy and dignity. With the understanding of the procedure and its implications, you can execute your parental authority responsibly and consciously decide the best for your child.

Informed consent involves several key elements:

1. Information: The healthcare professional is obligated to provide clear, complete, and factual information to aid your understanding.

2. Comprehension: It's essential that you comprehend the relevant information. If there are uncertainties, you must be able to question and receive satisfactory answers.

3. Voluntariness: The decision must be made voluntarily, free from external pressure or coercion.

4. Competence: You should be mentally capable of making decisions that significantly impact your child's health.

10.3. Preparing for the Vaccine Visit

Informed consent is a process, not a one-off conversation or signature. It begins the moment you're contemplating immunization for your child. Preparing ahead of the vaccine visit can facilitate a smooth and informed process.

1. Research: Start by conducting your research about the planned vaccines—the diseases they prevent, how they are administered, potential side effects, and the number of doses required.

2. Consult: Speak with your healthcare provider who can provide

more specific details based on your child's health condition.

3. Document: Make notes of any doubts, questions, or concerns that arise and bring these inquiries to your healthcare provider.

4. Discuss: Discuss the vaccines and the whole process with your child (if old enough to understand).

10.4. On the Day of the Vaccine Visit

It's essential that your healthcare provider explains the detailed process, including the particular vaccine(s) your child will be receiving, diseases being guarded against, potential risks, and benefits. You should also receive a Vaccine Information Sheet(VIS)–a document produced by the Centers for Disease Control and Prevention (CDC) for every vaccine licensed in the U.S.

Don't hesitate to ask questions or voice concerns—it's your right and responsibility. Your healthcare provider should respond with patience and comprehensiveness. Post this, you'll be required to sign an informed consent form. Ensure you are fully satisfied with the information before signing.

10.5. Post Vaccination: Monitoring and Recording

After the vaccination, observe your child closely for any adverse effects. While side effects are generally mild and temporary, it's crucial to report any severe ones to your healthcare provider immediately.

Keep a personal record of your child's vaccine history, including dates, vaccine names, and any side effects. It can be handy for future references and healthcare consultations.

10.6. Immunization: Empowerment through Consent

Informed consent empowers parents by involving them actively in their child's healthcare decisions, particularly immunizations. It supplements the understanding of vaccines, promoting their acceptance and uptake. However, remember that informed consent is just as significant each time your child receives a vaccine, as every vaccine and every circumstance may be different.

By providing informed consent, you are manifesting love and care for your child's health while actively contributing to a healthier society. Your role is vital—every informed decision moves us closer to a world free from preventable diseases.

Remember, your consent is more than a signature—it's a pledge towards a healthier future for your child and the community. In the sea of parenthood responsibilities, ensuring your child's immunization shines out as the beacon of their wellbeing and health.

Chapter 11. Looking Ahead: The Future of Vaccines and Immunization

The world of vaccines is an undeniably dynamic one. As scientists continue to unlock the mysteries of the human immune system, technological advancements and breakthroughs follow. Amidst these advancements on the horizon, we take a closer look at how vaccines and immunization work, shedding light on new developments and potential game-changers keen on attracting global attention.

11.1. The Mechanics of Vaccines and Immunization

Understanding how vaccines work is pivotal for appreciating prospective developments. The premise of vaccination is to stimulate the body's immune system to recognize and combat pathogens. To achieve this, certain elements of the pathogen, such as weakened or killed forms, proteins, or toxins, are introduced to our bodies via vaccines. This primes the immune system, creating a 'memory' of the pathogens, thereby facilitating a swift and efficient response when they encounter the actual pathogen in the future.

Yet, the constant evolution of pathogens and the rise of new diseases necessitate continuous research and development in vaccination. Consequently, the future of vaccines is likely to witness some innovative transformations.

11.2. Sub-Unit Vaccines: The Flight to a Safer Future

Traditional forms of vaccines use small amounts of live, attenuated (weakened) or inactivated (killed) disease-causing organisms to stimulate an immune response. However, contemporary and future vaccines have started to focus on using just a piece of the pathogen - essentially the proteins or sugars on their surface - rather than the whole organism. These are known as sub-unit vaccines.

Sub-unit vaccines offer a safer route to immunity. They are generally associated with fewer adverse effects since they exclude unnecessary constituents of the pathogen, leaving only essential antigens. These approaches can be fine-tuned to target specific strains or aspects of a disease, paving the way for highly specialized vaccinations.

11.3. The DNA and RNA Revolution

The race to develop a COVID-19 vaccine led to the notable breakthrough of mRNA vaccines by Pfizer-BioNTech and Moderna. Unlike traditional vaccines which introduce the pathogen components into the body, mRNA vaccines teach our cells to create a harmless piece of the protein unique to the pathogen. Our immune system then learns to recognize and defend against this protein, securing immunity against future invasions.

These innovative mRNA vaccines offer numerous future possibilities. They potentially phend off an array of diseases, from cancer to genetic disorders. Against the backdrop of rapid, large-scale production and adaptable design, these vaccines hold promise for the future of global disease control.

Similarly, DNA vaccines, although still in preliminary stages, have a promising future. These vaccines use genetically engineered DNA to provoke an immune response. Once inside, cells read this DNA 'recipe' and produce the pathogen's protein. Adjacent immune cells activate, recognizing and remembering how to fight this protein in case of a real confrontation.

11.4. Personalized Vaccines: The Era of Tailored Defense

Until recently, one-size-fits-all vaccines were commonly accepted. But the growing understanding of genetic variations and their effects on immunity has tilted the focus towards personalized vaccines that cater to individual immunity profiles.

In the future, we may see more custom-made vaccines, especially with the advent of genome sequencing and other genetic technologies. These allow for greater precision and effectiveness, particularly for diseases that show different strains in different regions or populations.

11.5. Vaccine Delivery: Strategies for the Next Generation

The traditional mode of vaccine delivery is through injections. However, ongoing research is exploring novel, more friendly modes of delivery, such as nasal sprays, oral pills, and patches.

Alternative delivery methods not only have the potential to increase vaccine coverage but also provide logistical benefits. Suppose the conventional 'cold-chain' transportation, a significant challenge for immunization programs in less developed regions, could be bypassed. In that case, vaccines could reach more remote regions, paving the way for enhanced global health security.

As we look ahead, the convergence of research, technology, and innovation marks an exciting new chapter in vaccines and global health. We might witness vaccines with an increased safety profile, personalized vaccines, novel vaccine delivery methods, and brand-new ways to provoke immune responses. The future might harbor challenges, but with scientific collaboration, we are armed with the tools to make strides in enhancing global health security.